- **50** -

Sensible

Weight Loss Tips

To **Melt Pounds**

Without Dieting

- **50** -

Sensible

Weight Loss Tips

To **Melt Pounds**

Without Dieting

by
Katherin Scott, A.Cht.

Wake-Up 2 Weight Loss

*Consciously creating a healthy body
and quality life*

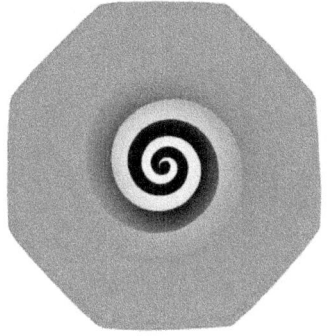

Wake-Up 2 Weight Loss

*Consciously creating a healthy body
and quality life*

Table of Contents

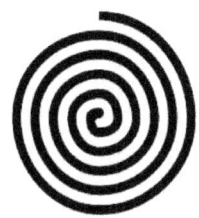

"Awareness is where meaning happens. If you want to change your body, a change in awareness must come first."

- **Depak Chopra**, Best-selling author of *Reinvent the Body, Resurrect the Soul*

Is your

lifestyle making

you fat?

Is your lifestyle making you fat?

Your habits, your beliefs, even your thoughts may be making and keeping you fat.

Isn't it time for you to WAKE-UP and consciously create the healthy body and quality life you desire and deserve?

Of course it is!

Now you CAN have the healthy body at your ideal weight *and* the quality life you've always dreamed of *and* with ease.

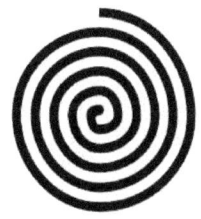

"If worry were an effective weight loss program, women would be invisible."

- **Nancy Drew**, Fictional, young amateur detective.

Hypnosis for

Weight Loss.

Really!

Hypnosis for Weight Loss. Really?

HYPNOSIS can help you to not only change your attitudes and habits around food and your ability to lose weight, it can also help you address and reframe the issues which contribute to unhealthy weight gain in the first place.

Learn to easily and effortlessly reprogram your subconscious mind and finally achieve the results you want and deserve!

It's time for you to Wake-Up 2 Weight Loss!

It's Your Time to
WAKE-UP 2
WEIGHT LOSS

Increase your awareness, heighten your ability to concentrate and stay focused, build your self-esteem and overcome fears and anxieties – it's easy with the power of hypnosis!

Imagine the healthy body you will have and quality life you will experience when you have all of these traits going for you.

Start Now!

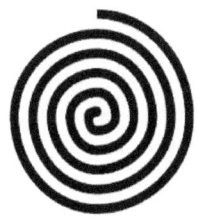

"*To become different from what we are, we must have some **awareness** of what we are.*"

- **Eric Hoffer**, Presidential Medal of Freedom recipient and author of *The Ordeal of Change*

- 50 -

Sensible

Weight Loss Tips

To **Melt Pounds**

Without Dieting

50 TIPS

1 Get your zzz's.

A lack of restful, restorative sleep can cause you to gain weight. A study published in the American Journal of Epidemiology confirmed that women who sleep less than seven hours a night were at an increased risk for weight gain and obesity. Another study in the Journal of Clinical Nutrition found that people who slept only five and a half hours a night ate 221 calories more than people who slept for eight and a half hours.

> "Hypnosis can actually **help you lose weight.**"
>
> - Jean Fain, Psychotherapist, Harvard Medical School

2 Practice positive self-talk.

Whether you are aware of it or not, you have a mental tape running constantly in your head; your self-talk, and it affects your moods and ultimately, your behavior. When these thoughts are negative or confining, they undermine your ability to change and ultimately get what you want. Practice more positive self-talk, telling yourself what a great job you are doing, how healthy you are eating and how you will fit into the next smaller size soon.

"Our food should be our medicine and our medicine should be our food."

- Hippocrates

3 Focus on high-quality calories.

A 200 calorie candy bar does not give your body the same nutrition as a 200 calorie bowl of lentil soup. And quality calories will help rev up your metabolism in a healthy way.

 Downsize your dinnerware.

Research shows that the bigger your bowl or plate, the more you will eat. Use smaller utensils too, such as smaller spoons, when eating.

 Count to 20.

One study found that diners with higher body mass indexes (BMIs) chewed each bite only 12 times compared with an average of fifteen times for healthy-weight people. Chewing your food more also makes your food taste sweeter as saliva has an enzyme called amylase that breaks down simple carbohydrates, such as in potatoes or wheat, into sugar.

*"Middle age is when you choose your cereal for the **fiber,** not the toy.."*

- Anonymous

Fill-up with fiber.

Fiber moves through your body more slowly than highly processed foods, making you feel full faster and satisfied longer. And recent studies show the more fiber you eat, the less you tend to weigh. Good sources of fiber are black beans, chickpeas, avocado and dried plums.

Workout in the morning.

A study in The Journal of Physiology finds that exercising first thing in the morning and before you eat breakfast can help you trim down faster. Breaking a sweat on an empty stomach in the morning improves glucose tolerance which spurs your body to shed fat.

Ask for a "to go" bag

at the start of your meal when eating in restaurants. By dividing your meal into what you will eat and what you will save for later, the temptation to clean your plate is eliminated.

Share your meal

with your spouse or friend when eating out. Many restaurants today serve large portion sizes. Enjoy the company, save money and eat a healthy portion size all at once.

 Sip some tea.

A study in The American Journal of Clinical Nutrition reveals that women with the highest intake of catechins, antioxidants in tea that may accelerate fat burn, gained less weight over 14 years than those with lower intakes. Green and white teas were found to have the most catechins.

> *"With weight loss the evidence is conclusive...* ***hypnosis does help people reduce."***
>
> *- Smithsonian Magazine*

11 Practice self-hypnosis.

Spend time every day visualizing yourself eating and enjoying healthy meals, fitting into slimming clothes, being of your ideal body weight. Listen to hypnosis CDs daily to program your mind for success.

> *"Take twice as long to eat half as much."*
>
> *- Anonymous*

12 Survey the buffet table

before you even pick up a plate. Look at everything that is available to eat then make the conscious choice of foods you are going to enjoy.

13 Get tested.

Have your doctor check your thyroid and hormone levels. Low thyroid levels can impair self-control and low levels of testosterone and DHEA are associated with obesity.

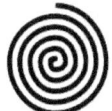

14 Change-it-up.

Your body burns fewer calories when it gets more efficient. Therefore, vary your workout to prevent boredom and to keep your body from getting too efficient in any one activity.

"In hypnosis, you can attain significant psycho-physiologic changes."

- Dr. Daniel Handel,
National Institute of Health

15 Think your way thin.

Visualizing your workout can help you trim, a study finds. Start by picturing your sneakers, as concrete objects are easier to visualize. Next, imagine all of the calories you are burning as you see yourself running in your mind's eye, noticing how easily and effortlessly you are shedding excess fat. Then see yourself reaching the finish line and notice how invigorated and proud you are as you complete your routine.

> *"To eat is a necessity, but to eat intelligently is an art."*
>
> *- La Rochefoucauld*

Read nutritional labels.

Check the fine print on the ingredient list. The shorter the list usually indicates a more nutritious and slimming pick whereas hard to pronounce ingredients are more likely artificial and not waist-friendly.

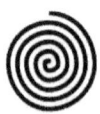

17 Read product labels frequently.

Manufacturers continually change their ingredients. Get into the habit of routinely reading labels to ensure you are still buying the product ingredients you desire to eat and thought were in the product.

"Don't eat anything your great-great grandmother wouldn't recognize as food."

- Michael Pollan, author of The Omnivore's Dilemma

18 Avoid "anti-nutrition" foods

such as trans fats, high-fructose corn syrup or potentially harmful food additives. These can spike your appetite and cause you to eat even more.

19 Use chopsticks.

Even if you are adept at using them, they may help you to slow down your food consumption so you will feel full without eating more. No chopsticks? Eat with your fork in your non-dominant hand to slow down your dexterity and the speed with which you shovel food into your mouth.

20 Eat more veggies.

Tufts University researchers found that the more veggies people eat, the thinner they are.

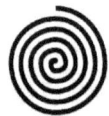

21 Switch to plain, un-sweetened yogurt.

Add your own fruit and a touch of cinnamon for a fresh taste. You will get the health benefits from the yogurt's probiotics without the unwanted sugar.

[26]

22 Pack your own healthy snacks

and avoid the vending machines. Fresh fruit, nuts, veggies, low fat cheese and unsweetened yogurt are good considerations and easy to carry with you.

23 Make healthy substitutions,

saving calories and adding flavor. Spaghetti squash and shredded zucchini are excellent substitutes for pasta as are vinegar and citrus fruits instead of cream sauces.

24 Beware of products labeled "fat-free".

Fat-free does not mean calorie-free and some people tend to over-indulge with "lower-fat" foods believing you can eat twice as much without having any repercussions in your weight or metabolism. Check the nutritional label before you indulge and, for truly fat-free, eat fruits and vegetables.

25 Enjoy your favorite dips;

salsa, hummus or guacamole – with veggies instead of chips or crackers. You'll save calories and consume fewer unhealthy oils.

26 Stop eating 2-3 hours before bed time

suggests Mark Hyman M.D. author of *Ultrametabolism*. Give your body the time it needs to digest the food.

> *"Alcohol is a diuretic, and the pounding headaches and furry tongue are caused by dehydration, so replacing the lost fluids is essential."*
>
> *- Anonymous*

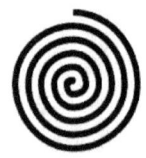

27 Avoid drinking your calories.

A recent study found that on average, Americans drink 450 calories a day, twice as many as we did thirty years ago. Just an extra 225 calories a day will put 23 pounds of fat a year on your body.

28 Choose fruit over fruit juice.

The fruit has fiber, which slows down the absorption of the natural sugars and keeps your blood sugar from spiking. You will also consume fewer calories when you eat the fruit.

29 Recognize dehydration vs. hunger.

Many people confuse being dehydrated with being hungry. Drink a glass of water first and then if you are still feeling hungry, eat. Research from Virginia Tech revealed drinking two cups of H2O before meals helped people lose five pounds more than those who said no to water.

30 Sit far away from the buffet

table and never face it when eating. Cornell University Food and Brand Lab researchers found that fatter diners tend to sit closer to the buffet and return more often for more helpings than slimmer people.

"Awareness is empowering."

- Rita Wilson, Actor

31 Write down everything you eat BEFORE

you put it into your mouth. This action creates awareness rather than mindlessly eating whatever is put in front of you.

32 Steer clear of processed foods.

A groundbreaking new study found that unprocessed meals take about 65 extra calories to digest compared with processed meals. Multiply that by three meals a day and you'll get a "bonus" burn of 1,365 calories per week.

> *"When you nourish your body with pure energy, you transform from the inside out."*
>
> *- Bill Phillips*

33 Find ways to move more.

Pace while you are talking on the phone. Take the stairs instead of the elevator. Scrub your floors. Make love with your partner. All of these activities burn calories and rev up your metabolism.

34 Get your Zen on.

Learn to meditate. Meditation has been found to boost the prefrontal cortex area of your brain resulting in greater self-control.

35 Face the truth.

Take an honest assessment of your waist-to-height ratio and your body mass index (BMI) so you will make healthy choices without being in denial.

36 Conquer your cravings.

Take natural supplements daily to reduce your cravings. Alpha-lipoic acid, chromium, L-glutamine, DL-phenylalanine, and N-acetyl-cysteine have all been found to be helpful.

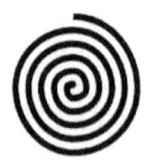

Choose healthy friends.

People tend to eat more when the people around them do too. Eat with people who share your healthy lifestyle rather than those who have bad eating habits.

38 Measure your progress.

According to research from the Minneapolis Heart Institute Foundation, people who weighed themselves at least weekly lost more weight than those who didn't. Spotting scale swings early allows you to tweak your eating and exercise routine before pounds can pile on. Its best to weigh at the same time each day to increase your measurement reliability.

> *"Your body is the baggage you must carry through life. The more excess the baggage, the shorter the trip."*
>
> *- Arnold H. Glasgow*

Savor your food.

Eating slowly and steadily can help you stay slim. According to a study in The Journal of Clinical Endocrinology and Metabolism, people who took 30 minutes to eat a dessert created more fullness hormones than those who ate faster.

Subdue your stress.

Under any physical or psychological stress, the body is designed to protect itself. It pumps hormones into your system that increase blood fats, sugar and insulin to prepare you for fight or flight, thereby causing you to store calories and conserve weight (just in case you need that energy reserve to run from a predator). Stress alone will cause weight gain, even without eating more or exercising less.

41 Pace yourself.

Multiple studies recommend spacing out your meals at regular intervals and keeping them all at about the same size. Eating meals at regular intervals has been linked to greater calorie burning after eating, lower fasting blood cholesterol levels, and better response to insulin. So if your goal is to eat 1600 calories daily, eating four 400 calorie meals, evenly spaced throughout the day would be a healthy plan.

"Health is the true wealth."

- Katherin Scott, A.Cht.

Eat smaller, more frequent meals.

In his book "Body Confidence," Mark Hyman M.D. suggests eating smaller meals every 3-4 hours to keep blood sugar levels balanced and to prevent overeating.

43 Sit down when you eat.

A study in the Journal of the American Dietetic Association found that 59 percent of young women eat on the go and on-the run eaters consume more total fat as well as more soda and fast food.

44 Eat healthy fats at mealtimes.

An Australian study showed that eating a meal with healthy fats, such as olive oil, significantly increased a person's fat-burning rate five hours later, particularly in people with more abdominal fat.

45 Cook at home whenever possible.

When you prepare your own meals from scratch, you are in charge of the ingredients and portion size.

46 Recognize portion sizes.

Huge portions, all-you-can-eat-buffets, and extra-large "single servings" of snack foods can all contribute to overeating. Learn about portion sizes:

a three-ounce serving of meat of poultry is about the size of a deck of cards or bar of soap, one serving of rice or pasta is the size of a tennis ball, a bread serving is the size of a CD case, and one serving of cheese is about the size of four dice.

 Set the table.

Studies suggest that the less distracted and stressed you are when you eat, the more efficiently your body absorbs nutrition. Eat at the table and focus on enjoying your food.

 Join the breakfast club.

If you're inclined to skip your morning meal, it's time to rethink that habit. The American Journal of Clinical Nutrition reveals that lifelong breakfast eaters have a waistline about two inches smaller than those of breakfast skippers. Plus, a morning meal may rev-up your metabolism.

Say NO to fried and breaded poultry.

Choose grilled or baked meats instead and cut at least 100 calories per serving.

Stop eating when you feel full.

Save the rest for later. This one habit can cut hundreds of calories from your daily intake of food.

"Those who think they have no time for healthy eating will sooner or later have to find time for illness."

- Edward Stanley

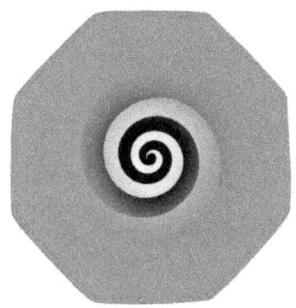

Wake-Up 2 Weight Loss

and consciously create a healthy
body and quality life.

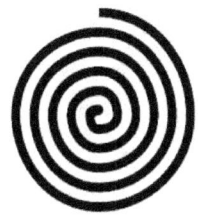

"When it becomes obvious that the goals cannot be reached, don't adjust the goals, adjust the action steps."

- **Confucius**, teacher, philosopher and political theorist, 551-479 BC

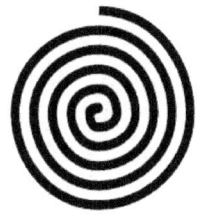

*"... **hypnosis** is not mind control. It's a naturally occurring state of concentration; it's **a means of enhancing your control over both your mind and your body**."*

\- **Dr. David Spiegel**,
Assoc. Chair of Psychiatry,
Stanford University School of Medicine

10 Ways to JUMP START your Weight Loss Plan Now!

10 Ways to JUMP START Your Weight Loss Plan Now!

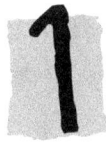 Download your FREE copy of the "**Love Yourself" Hypnosis CD** at www.LovingYouMP3.com.

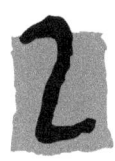 Discover the "**7 Surprising Things Making Your Fat and What to Do About Them"** by visiting www. WakeUp2WeightLoss.com

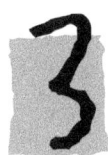 Write down five things you appreciate about your body right now in your copy of the Wake-Up 2 Weight Loss **Appreciation Journal.**

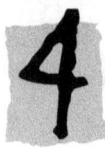 Call a friend and tell them that you've made the decision to consciously create a healthy body and quality life starting today.

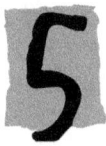 Remove five unhealthy foods from your pantry.

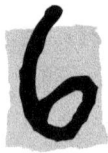 Visualize your body at your perfect weight for ten seconds, feeling healthy and happy.

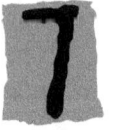 Find a picture that motivates you to stay on track with your goal of being at your ideal weight.

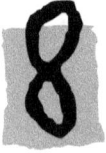 Mail yourself a hand-written note listing your specific goals and action steps for consciously creating a

healthy body and quality life.

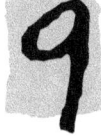 Move your body for 30 seconds right now. Stretch, dance, jog in place – whatever feels good to you.

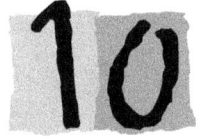 Celebrate your decision to start now! Woo-hoo!

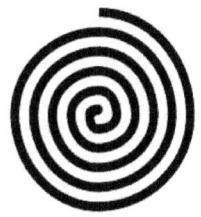

"Success is the sum of small efforts, repeated day in and day out."

- **Robert Collier**, Best-selling author of *The Secret of the Ages*

Meet the Founder
& Program Facilitator

of

Wake-Up 2
Weight Loss

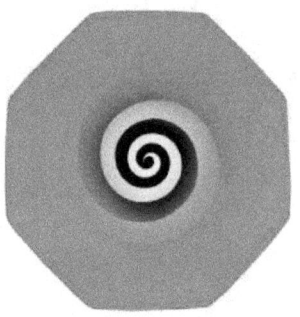

Katherin Scott is an expressive women who has experienced the ups and downs, the joys and disappointments, and the full-out sensation of life.

Katherin earned a degree in dietetics and is a Certified Advanced Clinical Hypnotherapist and NLP Practitioner from the Minnesota Institute of Hypnosis and Hypnotherapy.

With over a decade of teaching this Weight Loss with Hypnosis and NLP program to thousands of eager participants, Katherin is very excited to offer these sensible weight loss tips for you and invite you to join the Wake-Up 2 Weight Loss community.

Founder

Katherin Scott

Wake-Up 2
Weight Loss
Founder

KATHERIN SCOTT

"The power of visualization and self-hypnosis is mind-expanding – literally!"
- Katherin Scott

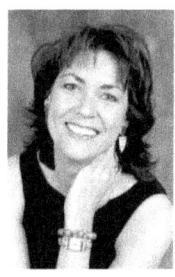

Guiding people beyond burnout to brilliance with every move they make is Katherin Scott's mission as a sought after keynote speaker, workshop leader and best-selling author.

As an impactful coach and hypnotherapist, Katherin shows people how to take specific, decisive steps forward to apply lessons that can have immediate and favorable effect on their life.

[53]

Her clients and seminar participants regularly report game-changing shifts in behavior that immediately translate to their health, relationships and even their paychecks.

Katherin is known for her energetic and enthusiastic presentation style and her disarming authenticity and warmth. She consistently delivers engaging, practical messages that compel audiences from 10 to 5,000 people to think differently about every move they make.

To engage Katherin,
send email to

**Katherin@
WakeUp2WeightLoss.com**

or call her office at
425-681-2620.

Also visit
www.Date2MateSecrets.com

Use HYPNOSIS

for Proven

Results!

Proven Results with the Wake-Up 2 Weight Loss Program

This is not your typical hypnosis for weight loss system.

Wake-Up 2 Weight Loss is a proven, mathematically based, powerful yet simple 3-step CUSTOMIZABLE program scientifically researched and developed by the Minnesota Institute of Hypnosis and Hypnotherapy.

Thousands have benefitted from this program nationwide losing, on average, 19 pounds and three inches in approximately 8 weeks.

Will power, goals, fad diets and a positive mental attitude are not enough to take inches off.

This program will take you through the process of re-programming your mind so you can create new stimulus responses to food, hunger urges, locations and unconscious reasons for eating.

The program addresses the CORE REASONS that weight is staying on the body and it will not change until the two key mental programs start running differently.

Now you can begin to feel better as you realize that your weight will begin to fade away... giving yourself a new sense of pride and a slimmer look ... a healthy body and a quality life.

Even if you've never been able to lose weight before, you're more likely to now succeed with hypnosis.

Experience this powerful program for yourself, customized specifically for you. Join the Wake-Up 2 Weight Loss community!

Visit www.WakeUp2Weightloss.com and download your *free* report **"7 Surprising Things Making You Fat and What To Do About Them"**.

Wishing you much love and happiness,

Katherin

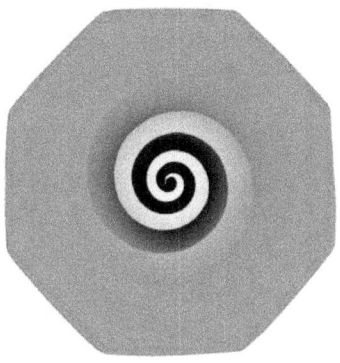

Wake-Up 2 Weight Loss

and consciously create a healthy body and quality life.

NOTES:

NOTES:

NOTES:

www.ingramcontent.com/pod-product-compliance
Lightning Source LLC
Chambersburg PA
CBHW060217290526
45789CB00003B/1304